D1526202

KETTLEBELL WORKOUT

FOR SENIORS

Revitalize Your Golden Years: Unleashing Strength, Flexibility, and Vitality with Safe and Effective Kettlebell Exercises for seniors

AUDREY GLEASON

TABLE OF CONTENTS

INTRODUCTION

Dear Senior Friend,

Welcome to an exciting new chapter in your fitness journey! I'm thrilled to guide you through the invigorating world of kettlebell workouts. Whether you're new to exercise or a seasoned fitness enthusiast, embracing kettlebell training at this age opens up a realm of possibilities for enhancing your strength, flexibility, and vitality.

Kettlebell workouts hold a special allure for seniors like yourself. They offer a dynamic and engaging way to stay active while reaping numerous health benefits. Unlike traditional gym machines, kettlebells provide a versatile and functional approach to strength training, catering to the unique needs and abilities of older adults.

As you embark on this journey, let me share with you the incredible benefits awaiting you:

1. Strength and Stability: Kettlebell exercises target multiple muscle groups simultaneously, helping you build strength and improve stability. By enhancing your muscle mass and coordination, you'll find everyday tasks become easier, from lifting groceries to navigating stairs with confidence.

2. *Flexibility and Mobility:* Aging often brings stiffness and reduced range of motion. However, kettlebell workouts incorporate dynamic movements that promote flexibility and mobility. You'll discover newfound freedom in your joints, allowing you to move more comfortably and gracefully.

3. *Cardiovascular Health:* Don't let age be a barrier to cardiovascular fitness! Kettlebell training offers a cardio boost through exercises like swings and circuits, elevating your heart rate and enhancing circulation. Improved cardiovascular health means more energy for enjoying your favorite activities and adventures.

4. *Mental Wellbeing:* Physical activity is a powerful antidote to stress and anxiety, and kettlebell workouts are no exception. As you engage in each exercise, you'll experience a sense of focus and mindfulness, leaving you feeling energized and uplifted. Exercise has the remarkable ability to boost mood and promote mental clarity, enriching your overall quality of life.

Now, let me introduce you to some inspirational seniors who have experienced the transformative power of kettlebell training:

"At 67, I never imagined I'd be swinging kettlebells like a pro! Not only have I gained strength and vitality, but I've also discovered a newfound sense of empowerment. Age truly is just a number when you have the right tools and mindset." - *Patricia*

"After retiring, I was looking for a way to stay active and engaged. Kettlebell workouts have become the highlight of my day! Not only do I feel stronger and more agile, but I've also made new friends at the gym. It's never too late to start living your best life!" - *Robert*

These individuals, like many others, have embraced the kettlebell journey with open arms and reaped the rewards. Now, it's your turn to experience the joy and fulfillment that comes from investing in your health and wellbeing.

Benefits of Kettlebell Workouts for You

As you embark on this journey, let's explore the myriad benefits awaiting you, designed to enhance your strength, balance, flexibility, and cardiovascular health. These benefits are not just promises but proven outcomes supported by scientific research and the inspiring stories of fellow seniors like yourself who have experienced remarkable transformations.

1. Improved Strength and Muscle Tone

You'll be amazed at how kettlebell workouts can revitalize your muscles, enhancing your strength and muscle tone. By engaging in these exercises, you'll target multiple muscle groups simultaneously, leading to increased muscle mass and functional strength. Imagine feeling more capable and confident in your daily activities, whether it's carrying groceries or playing with your grandchildren. With every swing and press, you're building a foundation of strength that empowers you to live life to the fullest.

2. Enhanced Balance and Stability

Maintaining your balance and stability becomes easier as you incorporate kettlebell workouts into your routine. These dynamic exercises challenge your coordination and proprioception, helping you stay steady on your feet and reducing the risk of falls. Picture yourself navigating uneven terrain with ease and grace, knowing that your newfound stability is keeping you safe and secure. With each balanced movement, you're building a solid foundation for a vibrant and active lifestyle.

3. Increased Flexibility and Range of Motion

Bid farewell to stiffness and limited mobility as you embrace kettlebell training. The dynamic nature of these exercises promotes flexibility and joint mobility, allowing you to move more freely and comfortably. Say hello to reaching higher, bending lower, and moving with greater ease. Whether it's reaching for a high shelf or tying your shoelaces, you'll experience newfound freedom in your movements, enhancing your overall quality of life.

4. Cardiovascular Conditioning

Your heart will thank you as you engage in kettlebell workouts that elevate your cardiovascular health. These exercises offer an effective way to get your heart pumping and improve your aerobic capacity. Picture yourself with more energy and vitality, tackling activities with renewed vigor and enthusiasm. With each swing and lift, you're boosting your heart health and enhancing your endurance, paving the way for a more active and fulfilling lifestyle.

5. Bone Density and Osteoporosis Prevention

Protecting your bones and preventing osteoporosis becomes a priority as you age, and kettlebell training can help you achieve just that. These weight-bearing exercises stimulate bone growth and increase bone mineral density, reducing the risk of fractures. Imagine feeling stronger and more resilient, knowing that your bones are fortified against the effects of aging. With each rep and set, you're investing in your long-term bone health and vitality.

6. Management of Arthritis and Joint Pain

If arthritis and joint pain have been holding you back, kettlebell workouts offer a gentle yet effective solution. These low-impact exercises help alleviate stiffness, increase joint lubrication, and strengthen surrounding muscles. Picture yourself moving with greater ease and comfort, enjoying activities without the burden of pain. With each controlled movement, you're reclaiming your mobility and independence, proving that age is no obstacle to an active and fulfilling life.

7. Cognitive Function and Mental Wellbeing

Lastly, let's not forget the profound impact of kettlebell training on your cognitive function and mental wellbeing. Physical activity has been shown to enhance brain health and reduce the risk of cognitive decline. As you engage in these exercises, you'll experience improved focus, clarity, and mood. Imagine feeling more alert and engaged, with a sense of accomplishment and joy after each workout. With each swing and press, you're nurturing not just your body but also your mind, ensuring a vibrant and fulfilling life as you age gracefully.

Safety Considerations and Precautions

As we embark on your kettlebell journey, safety is paramount. Before diving into any new exercise program, especially as a senior, it's crucial to consult with your doctor or healthcare professional. Your safety and wellbeing are our top priorities, and understanding your unique medical needs and limitations will guide us in crafting a safe and effective fitness plan tailored just for you.

Consulting Your Doctor

Before picking up a kettlebell or engaging in any physical activity, schedule a consultation with your doctor to discuss your fitness goals and any pre-existing medical conditions. Your doctor can provide valuable insights and recommendations based on your health history, ensuring that your exercise program is both safe and beneficial. Together, we'll work as a team to create a plan that supports your health and wellbeing every step of the way.

Choosing the Right Weight

Selecting the appropriate weight for your kettlebell is crucial for preventing injury and maximizing the effectiveness of your workouts. As a general guideline, choose a weight that allows you to perform each exercise with proper form and technique while still challenging your muscles. Start with a lighter weight and gradually increase as you become more comfortable and proficient. Remember, it's always better to start conservatively and progress gradually rather than risking injury by lifting too heavy too soon.

Warm-Up and Cool-Down Routines

Before diving into your kettlebell workout, take the time to properly warm up your muscles and prepare your body for exercise. A dynamic warm-up consisting of movements like arm circles, leg swings, and hip circles can help increase blood flow, improve flexibility, and reduce the risk of injury. After your workout, don't forget to cool down with some gentle stretches to help relax your muscles and promote recovery.

Listening to Your Body

Above all, listen to your body and honor its signals. Pay attention to how you feel during exercise and avoid pushing through pain or discomfort. If something doesn't feel right, stop immediately and reassess your form or reduce the weight. It's important to challenge yourself, but not at the expense of your safety and wellbeing. Remember, progress is a journey, and consistency is key. Trust the process, be patient with yourself, and celebrate every step forward on your path to better health and fitness.

Now, let's pick up those kettlebells and embark on this adventure together, one safe and confident rep at a time!

With dedication to your wellbeing,

-Audrey

Your Professional Gym Instructor

I

UNDERSTANDING KETTLEBELL

In the realm of fitness, there exists a timeless tool that has endured centuries of evolution and innovation—the kettlebell. Its origins trace back to the depths of history, where strength, endurance, and tradition intersect. This humble piece of equipment has found its place in modern fitness routines, but its journey spans far beyond contemporary gyms.

Ancient Beginnings: The Birth of Kettlebells

Our journey commences in ancient Russia, where the kettlebell's story first unfolds. Historians suggest that kettlebells originated in the 18th century, emerging as a training tool for Russian strongmen known as *"Gireviks."* These early kettlebells, resembling cannonballs with handles, were crafted from cast iron and served as a testament to the ingenuity of their creators.

The term *"girevoy sport"* encapsulates the essence of early kettlebell training, as athletes showcased their prowess through a series of dynamic movements. These exercises not only cultivated strength but also fostered resilience and agility—a testament to the multifaceted nature of kettlebell workouts.

As time marched forward, the influence of kettlebell training transcended borders, captivating audiences far beyond the shores of Russia. In the 20th century, kettlebells found their way into Soviet military training programs, where they became instrumental in honing the physical prowess of soldiers.

Yet, it was not solely the domain of the military elite; kettlebells permeated diverse spheres of society, from athletes seeking peak performance to everyday individuals pursuing functional fitness. This widespread adoption bore witness to the versatility and efficacy of kettlebell workouts, cementing their status as a staple in the realm of strength training.

Fast forward to the 21st century, where a fitness renaissance breathed new life into age-old practices. Kettlebell training experienced a resurgence, propelled by the growing popularity of functional fitness and unconventional training modalities.

Fitness enthusiasts, athletes, and trainers alike embraced kettlebells as a means to challenge convention and unlock new dimensions of physical performance. The simplicity of the kettlebell belied its transformative potential, offering a gateway to strength, endurance, and mobility.

Central to the revitalization of kettlebell training were pioneering figures who championed its virtues and shared their expertise with the world. Among these luminaries, Pavel Tsatsouline stands out as a trailblazer whose contributions helped propel kettlebells into the mainstream.

Through his writings, workshops, and instructional videos, Pavel demystified kettlebell training, making it accessible to novices and seasoned athletes alike. His emphasis on technique, consistency, and the principle of "hardstyle" forged a path for practitioners to maximize their gains while minimizing the risk of injury.

Furthermore, Pavel's collaboration with Dragon Door Publications catalyzed the dissemination of kettlebell knowledge, spawning a wealth of resources that empowered individuals to embark on their own kettlebell journey.

In the contemporary fitness landscape, kettlebell training continues to evolve, embracing innovation while honoring tradition. From the emergence of specialized kettlebell certifications to the integration of kettlebells into CrossFit and functional fitness regimens, the possibilities are limitless.

Moreover, the advent of competition kettlebells has ushered in a new era of standardized training protocols and competitive events. Organizations such as the International Kettlebell Sport Federation (IKSF) and the World Kettlebell Club (WKC) provide platforms for athletes to showcase their skills and vie for prestigious titles on the global stage.

Beyond their utility as a fitness tool, kettlebells have permeated popular culture, leaving an indelible mark on the zeitgeist. From viral workout videos to Hollywood blockbusters featuring ripped protagonists wielding kettlebells with aplomb, the imagery of kettlebell training resonates with audiences worldwide.

This cultural resonance speaks to the enduring appeal of kettlebell workouts, transcending mere exercise to embody a lifestyle characterized by strength, resilience, and determination.

THE ESSENTIAL: KETTLEBELL AND YOU

I know some exercise equipment might seem intimidating, but kettlebells are surprisingly user-friendly, and they offer a fantastic workout for people of all ages and abilities – especially us active seniors!

Think of them as a versatile, single weight that lets you work your whole body. They're a great way to build strength, improve balance, and boost your energy levels – all while having some fun!

Types and What's Right for You

There are three main types of kettlebells you might encounter:

Cast Iron: These are the classic kettlebells – the ones you might see in fitness magazines. They're super durable and come in a wide range of weights. However, they can be a bit pricey and might feel a little cold in your hands.

Vinyl: A good option for beginners like us! They're lighter and easier to handle, and the vinyl coating provides a good grip. Plus, they're quieter when you put them down (no clanging metal!). The downside? They usually come in a more limited weight range.

Adjustable: These clever kettlebells allow you to change the weight inside by adding or removing plates. A good option if you plan to progress quickly, but they can be a bit bulkier and more expensive than the others.

My recommendation for you? Start with vinyl! They're comfortable, affordable, and quieter, which is always a bonus. Plus, we'll focus on proper form over heavy weights, so a lighter option is perfect for learning the ropes.

Choosing Your Weight: Safety First!

Now, let's talk about weight selection. The most important thing to remember is to start light. It's much better to begin with a weight you can control comfortably and gradually increase it as you get stronger. Here's a good rule of thumb:

For beginners: Aim for a weight that feels challenging for 10-12 repetitions of an exercise. If you can easily do 15 repetitions, it's time to move up a weight.

Listen to your body: If you feel any pain or discomfort, stop the exercise and choose a lighter weight. Pain is never a good sign!

Remember, we're not powerlifters here. We want to focus on controlled movements and good form – that's where the real magic happens.

A Quick Anatomy Lesson

Now, let's take a closer look at the kettlebell itself. It might look a bit strange at first, but it's actually quite simple:

Handle: This is the part you grip. Look for a handle that's smooth and wide enough for a comfortable hold.

Body: This is the main weight of the kettlebell. It can be round, square, or even hexagonal. Don't worry too much about the shape – it won't affect your workout significantly.

Base: This is the flat bottom of the kettlebell that allows it to stand upright when you set it down.

There you have it! A basic breakdown of your new workout buddy. It might seem like a lot to take in at first, but trust me, kettlebells are surprisingly easy to learn and use.

In the next session, we'll start with some basic kettlebell exercises, focusing on proper form and technique. You'll be amazed at how quickly you can start feeling the benefits of this fantastic workout!

Just like when we were younger and played sports, warming up before and cooling down after your kettlebell workout is absolutely crucial. It might seem like an extra step, but trust me, these routines are your best friends for a safe and enjoyable exercise experience!

Why Warm-Up? It's All About Preparation

Think of your body like a well-oiled machine. Before you jump into a challenging workout, you need to get all the parts moving smoothly together. A proper warm-up helps to:

Increase your heart rate and blood flow: This prepares your cardiovascular system for the workout ahead, delivering oxygen and nutrients to your muscles for better performance.

Loosen up your joints: As we age, our bodies naturally become a little stiffer. Warming up your joints improves your range of motion and reduces the risk of injury.

Engage your core and improve stability: A good warm-up activates your core muscles, which are like your body's internal stabilizers. This helps you maintain proper form during your kettlebell exercises, reducing the risk of strain or falls.

Prepare your mind: Warming up gives your body and mind a chance to transition from everyday activities to a focused workout state. It helps you become mentally prepared for the exercises ahead.

Warm-Up Exercises for Seniors: Gentle Yet Effective

Here are some excellent dynamic stretches and mobility exercises perfect for seniors using kettlebells:

Arm circles: Stand with your feet shoulder-width apart and arms outstretched at shoulder height. Make small circles forward for 10 repetitions, then reverse direction for another 10.

Shoulder rolls: Gently roll your shoulders forward in a circular motion for 10 repetitions, then reverse direction for another 10.

Neck rolls: Slowly roll your head in a circular motion, leading with your chin. Do 5 repetitions in each direction.

Torso twists: Stand with your feet shoulder-width apart and arms extended to your sides. Gently twist your torso to the right as far as comfortably possible, hold for a second, then return to center. Repeat on the left side. Do 5 repetitions on each side.

Ankle circles: Sit in a chair and extend one leg straight out in front of you. Rotate your ankle in a small circular motion for 10 repetitions, then reverse direction for another 10. Repeat with the other leg.

Focus on controlled movements and listen to your body. If you feel any pain, stop the exercise and modify it as needed. Remember, we're aiming for gentle stretching, not pushing yourself to the limit.

Cool-Down: Rewarding Your Body for Hard Work

Now that you've completed your kettlebell workout, it's time to cool down and help your body recover. A good cool-down routine helps to:

Gradually lower your heart rate and blood flow: This allows your body to return to its resting state more smoothly.

Improve blood flow to remove waste products: Exercise creates lactic acid, which can contribute to muscle soreness. Cooling down helps flush out these waste products and reduces post-workout stiffness.

Maintain flexibility: Holding gentle stretches after your workout helps maintain the improved range of motion achieved during your warm-up.

A Gentle Cool-Down Routine for Seniors

Here's a simple cool-down routine you can do after your kettlebell workout:

Walking lunges: Take a big step forward with one leg, lowering your back knee until it nearly touches the ground. Push back up to standing and repeat with the other leg. Do 5-10 lunges on each side.

Hamstring stretch: Sit on the floor with your legs extended in front of you. Reach for your toes, keeping your back straight, and hold for a comfortable stretch for 15-30 seconds.

Quad stretch: Stand on one leg and grab the ankle of your other leg behind you. Gently pull your heel towards your buttocks until you feel a stretch in your quadriceps. Hold for 15-30 seconds, then repeat on the other side.

Cat-cow stretches: Get on your hands and knees with your back flat and neck in line with your spine. As you inhale, arch your back and look up (cow pose). As you exhale, round your back and tuck your chin to your chest (cat pose). Repeat 5-10 times.

Remember: Don't skip the warm-up and cool-down! These routines are essential for a safe and enjoyable kettlebell experience.

2

MASTERING YOUR MOVEMENT: FOUNDATIONAL EXERCISES

BODYWEIGHT EXERCISES FOR KETTLEBELL SUCCESS

Just like a sturdy house needs a solid base, your kettlebell workouts will benefit greatly from a foundation built with bodyweight exercises.

These exercises utilize your own body weight as resistance, making them perfect for beginners and seniors alike. They're a fantastic way to:

Improve overall strength and endurance: Bodyweight exercises target multiple muscle groups at once, building strength throughout your body. This improved strength will translate beautifully to your kettlebell routines later on.

Enhance balance and coordination: Many bodyweight exercises challenge your balance and require coordination. This not only helps with everyday activities but also improves your stability for more advanced exercises with kettlebells.

Increase bone density: Weight-bearing exercises like squats and lunges can help maintain bone density, which is especially important as we age.

Reduce your risk of injury: A strong body is a less injury-prone body. Building strength and stability with bodyweight exercises prepares your muscles and joints for the demands of kettlebell training.

Now, let's explore some fantastic bodyweight exercises that will get you prepped for your kettlebell adventure:

1. Squats (and Variations)

Squats are a fundamental exercise that works your legs, core, and glutes. Here's how to do them safely and effectively:

1. Stand with your feet shoulder-width apart, toes slightly pointed outward.
2. Keep your core engaged and back straight as you lower yourself down as if you're going to sit in a chair.
3. Bend your knees until your thighs are parallel to the ground (or as low as comfortably possible).
4. Push back through your heels to return to standing position.

Safety Considerations

Don't let your knees cave inward as you squat. Keep them tracking over your toes.

Focus on keeping your back straight and avoid hunching forward.

Hold onto a sturdy chair for balance if needed.

Variations

Chair Squats: A great way to build confidence. Stand in front of a chair with your back to it. Lower yourself down as if to sit, then push back up to standing.

Wall Squats: Stand with your back flat against a wall. Slide down the wall as if you're sitting, keeping your core engaged and back straight. Hold for a few seconds, then slide back up.

2. Lunges with Step-Ups

Lunges work your legs and core, while step-ups add a balance challenge. Here's how to do them:

1. Stand with your feet hip-width apart.
2. Step forward with one leg, lowering your body until both knees are bent at 90-degree angles.
3. Push back through your front heel to return to standing.

4. Repeat with the other leg.

For Step-Ups:

1. Find a sturdy step or bench that's comfortable for you.
2. Step up onto the platform with one leg, bringing your other knee up towards your chest.
3. Step back down and repeat with the other leg.

Safety Considerations

Keep your front knee tracking over your ankle as you lunge.

Don't let your back knee touch the ground during lunges.

Choose a step height that allows you to maintain good form.

3. Push-Ups (with Modifications)

Push-ups are a classic upper body exercise, but they can be challenging for some. Here are some modifications that still provide benefits:

Wall Push-Ups: Stand facing a wall with your feet shoulder-width apart. Place your hands flat on the wall at shoulder height. Lean into the wall and bend your elbows, lowering your chest towards the wall. Push back to straighten your arms.

Incline Push-Ups: Find a sturdy bench or countertop at a comfortable height. Perform push-ups with your hands placed on the surface, lowering your chest towards the bench.

Safety Considerations

Keep your core engaged and back straight throughout the push-up.

Don't let your lower back sag. Modify the height as needed to maintain proper form.

4. Rows (using Chairs or Resistance Bands)

Rows strengthen your back, shoulders, and biceps. Here are two options for you:

Chair Rows: Sit on a sturdy chair with your feet flat on the floor. Lean forward from your hips, keeping your back straight, and reach out with your arms (as if holding dumbbells). Row your arms back, squeezing your shoulder blades together, then extend your arms back out.

Resistance Band Rows: Secure a resistance band around a doorknob or sturdy object at waist height. Stand facing the doorknob with your feet shoulder-width apart. Hold the band taut with both hands, elbows bent and close to your body. Row your arms back, squeezing your shoulder blades together, then slowly extend your arms back out to the starting position.

Safety Considerations

Keep your back straight and avoid hunching over during rows.

Don't use a weight or resistance band that's too heavy. You should feel challenged but not strained.

The Importance of Proper Form

No matter which bodyweight exercise you choose, proper form is very important. Here are some general tips you should follow:

Focus on quality over quantity. It's better to do a few repetitions with perfect form than many with poor form.

Breathe properly. Inhale as you lower yourself down or extend your arms out, and exhale as you push back up or pull your arms in.

Move slowly and with control. Don't rush through the exercises.

Listen to your body. If you feel any pain, stop the exercise and rest.

Building a Bodyweight Routine

I have provided a sample bodyweight routine you can try 2-3 times per week below:

- ➢ Warm-up (5 minutes): Light cardio like walking or gentle stretches.
- ➢ Squats (or variations) - 3 sets of 10 repetitions
- ➢ Lunges (or step-ups) - 3 sets of 10 repetitions per leg
- ➢ Push-ups (modified if needed) - 3 sets of as many repetitions as comfortable
- ➢ Rows (chair or resistance band) - 3 sets of 10 repetitions

Bodyweight exercises are a fantastic way to build a strong foundation for your kettlebell workouts. They'll help you improve your overall strength, balance, and coordination, preparing you for more advanced movements with greater confidence and reduced risk of injury. So, embrace these exercises, feel the burn, and get ready to take your fitness to the next level with kettlebells!

Now that you've built a strong foundation with bodyweight exercises, it's time to go into the exciting world of kettlebell grips! Don't worry, these aren't complicated handshakes – they're simply different ways of holding the kettlebell to perform various exercises effectively and safely.

We are going to explore the three main kettlebell grips and how they're used:

1. Two-Handed Grips

This is the most basic and common grip used in many kettlebell exercises. Here's how to achieve a safe and strong two-handed grip:

1. Stand with your feet shoulder-width apart and the kettlebell resting on the floor in front of you.
2. Squat down and grasp the handle with both hands, thumbs wrapped around the outside.
3. Your knuckles should be facing white (pointing towards the ceiling) as you lift the kettlebell.

Maintaining Proper Posture

As you lift the kettlebell, keep your core engaged and back straight. Imagine a straight line running from your head down your spine.

Avoid arching your back or rounding your shoulders.

2. One-Handed Grips

One-handed grips add a new element of challenge and work your core stability even more. Here are two common variations:

Neutral Grip: Similar to the two-handed grip, but you hold the kettlebell with one hand, thumb wrapped around the outside of the handle.

Bottom-Up Grip: This grip requires the kettlebell to be held upside down. Wrap your fingers around the handle and rest your forearm on the body of the kettlebell.

Safety Considerations

One-handed exercises require good balance and coordination. Start with lighter weights until you feel comfortable.

Maintain a strong core and keep your back straight throughout the exercise.

3. Transitional Grips

These grips are used to switch between two-handed and one-handed exercises smoothly. Here's an example:

Clean Grip: This grip involves starting with the kettlebell on the floor and lifting it into a racked position (resting on your forearm). You use a two-handed grip to lift it, then transition to a one-handed neutral grip as you bring it up to your forearm.

Matching the Grip to the Exercise

The type of grip you use depends on the specific kettlebell exercise you're performing. Here's a breakdown for some common exercises:

Swings: Two-handed grip.

Goblet Squats: Two-handed grip or bottom-up grip.

Clean and Press: Transitional grip (clean) to neutral grip (press).

Rows: One-handed neutral grip.

Why is Grip So Important?

Using the correct grip is important for several reasons:

Safety: A proper grip ensures you have good control over the kettlebell, minimizing the risk of dropping it and injuring yourself.

Effectiveness: Using the right grip allows you to target the intended muscle groups more effectively during each exercise.

Injury Prevention: Maintaining a neutral spine and core engagement while using the correct grip helps prevent back strain or other injuries.

MASTERING THE BASIC MOVEMENTS

Now that you've built a solid foundation with bodyweight exercises and mastered the different kettlebell grips, it's time to explore the fundamental movements that will form the backbone of your kettlebell routine! These basic exercises target various muscle groups and can be combined to create a well-rounded workout.

Remember: Safety is paramount. Always start with lighter weights and prioritize proper form over heavy lifting. As your strength and confidence improve, you can gradually increase the weight. Here's a breakdown of four essential kettlebell movements:

1. The Swing

The swing is a dynamic exercise that works your legs, core, glutes, and shoulders. It's a fantastic way to improve overall fitness and power.

How to Do It

Stand with your feet shoulder-width apart, toes slightly pointed outward.

Hold the kettlebell with a two-handed grip (thumbs wrapped around the outside of the handle) between your legs, keeping your back straight and core engaged.

Hinge at your hips (not your knees) to send the kettlebell back between your legs. Keep your arms straight and shoulders down.

As the kettlebell swings back, feel your glutes and hamstrings engage to powerfully thrust your hips forward, naturally straightening your back. The momentum from your hips propels the kettlebell up to chest height (not above your shoulders).

Maintain a neutral spine throughout the movement. Avoid arching your back or rounding your shoulders.

Squeeze your glutes at the top of the swing before reversing the motion and hinging back down to the starting position.

Safety Considerations

Don't use your arms to lift the kettlebell. The power comes from your hips.

Keep your core engaged throughout the movement to protect your spine.

Don't swing the kettlebell above shoulder height.

2. The Goblet Squat

The goblet squat is a compound exercise that strengthens your legs, core, and upper back. It's a fantastic way to build lower body strength and improve balance.

How to Do It

Stand with your feet shoulder-width apart, holding the kettlebell vertically in front of your chest with a two-handed grip (thumbs wrapped around the outside of the handle).

Keep your elbows tucked in close to your body and core engaged.

Hinge at your hips and bend your knees as if you're going to sit in a chair. Lower down until your thighs are parallel to the ground (or as low as comfortably possible).

Push back through your heels to return to the standing position.

Safety Considerations

Keep your core engaged and back straight throughout the squat.

Don't let your knees cave inward as you squat. Keep them tracking over your toes.

Focus on maintaining proper form rather than how low you squat.

Variation

Bottom-Up Goblet Squat: This variation challenges your core stability even more. Hold the kettlebell upside down with your hand on the base and your forearm resting against the body of the kettlebell. Perform the squat as described above.

3. The Deadlift

The deadlift is a fundamental exercise that works your entire posterior chain (backside of your body), including your hamstrings, glutes, and lower back. It helps improve strength, posture, and balance.

How to Do It

Stand with your feet shoulder-width apart, toes slightly pointed outward.

The kettlebell should be resting on the floor in front of you.

Hinge at your hips and bend your knees slightly, keeping your back straight and core engaged. Reach down with both hands (thumbs wrapped around the outside of the handle) and grasp the kettlebell.

Maintain a flat back throughout the movement. Don't round your shoulders or arch your back.

Squeezing your glutes and hamstrings, slowly stand up straight, lifting the kettlebell along your body. Keep the kettlebell close to your legs throughout the movement.

Lower the kettlebell back down to the floor with control, reversing the hinge motion in your hips and keeping your back straight.

Safety Considerations

Don't use your back to lift the kettlebell. The power comes from your legs and glutes.

Keep your core engaged to protect your spine.

Don't round your back at any point during the movement.

Start with a very light weight to ensure proper form.

4. The Floor Press

The floor press is a variation of the traditional push-up that utilizes the kettlebell for added stability and core engagement. It strengthens your chest, shoulders, and triceps.

How to Do It

Start in a high plank position with your hands slightly wider than shoulder-width apart, holding a kettlebell in each hand with a neutral grip (thumbs wrapped around the outside of the handle). Your body should form a straight line from head to heels.

Engage your core and keep your back straight throughout the movement.

Lower your chest down towards the floor, bending your elbows at a 90-degree angle. Keep the kettlebells close to your body as you descend.

Push back through your palms to return to the starting position.

Safety Considerations

Don't let your lower back sag or arch your back during the press.

Modify the exercise by performing it on your knees if a full plank is too challenging.

Variation

Single-arm Floor Press: This variation challenges your core stability even more. Perform the floor press with one kettlebell at a time, holding the other hand behind your back for support.

The Importance of Starting Light

As we mentioned earlier, it's crucial to start with a lighter weight and focus on proper form. Here are some additional tips:

Choose a weight that allows you to perform 10-12 repetitions with good form. If you can easily do more than 12 repetitions, it's time to increase the weight slightly.

Don't be afraid to experiment with different weights to find what feels comfortable and challenging.

3

BUILDING STRENGTH AND POWER

Having mastered the basic kettlebell swing, you're ready to elevate your workout and tap into the power this exercise offers! Kettlebell swing variations are fantastic tools for seniors looking to build upper body strength and power while maintaining proper form and safety. These variations add new challenges to the swing, engaging more muscle groups and boosting your overall fitness potential.

Now, let's explore some exciting swing variations to add power to your routine:

1. Two-Handed Swings

While you've mastered the basic two-handed swing, let's refine it to build a strong foundation for power generation. Here's what to focus on:

Explosive Hip Hinge: Remember, the power comes from your hips, not your back. Focus on a powerful hip hinge at the bottom of the swing, squeezing your glutes and hamstrings to propel the kettlebell upwards. Think of pushing the floor away with your feet.

Core Engagement: A strong core is crucial for power transfer and stability. Brace your core throughout the movement, keeping your back straight and avoiding any twisting or arching.

Safety Considerations

Maintain a neutral spine throughout the swing.

Don't swing the kettlebell above shoulder height.

Keep your core engaged to protect your lower back.

2. Single-Arm Swings

Single-arm swings challenge your core stability even further, forcing your entire body to work together to maintain proper posture and control. Here's how to perform them with power:

Maintain Proper Posture: Stand tall with a neutral spine and core engaged. Don't let your hips twist or your back round as you swing the kettlebell.

Explosive Hip Drive: Similar to the two-handed swing, focus on a powerful hip hinge to initiate the movement. Drive with your hips to propel the kettlebell upwards, engaging your core to maintain stability.

Safety Considerations:

Start with a lighter weight than you use for two-handed swings.

Focus on controlled movements – avoid jerking the kettlebell.

Maintain proper posture throughout the swing, especially with your core engaged.

3. High Pulls

The high pull is a fantastic variation that builds explosive power in your upper body while still incorporating the core and lower body engagement of the swing. Here's how to unleash your inner power with proper technique:

Explosive Hip Hinge: Initiate the movement with a powerful hip hinge, just like in the other swing variations.

Explosive Pull: As the kettlebell swings up to chest height, explosively pull it upwards with your arms, bringing it close to your body and finishing with your elbows bent at a 90-degree angle beside your head. Imagine catching the kettlebell in your hand.

Lower with Control: Reverse the movement with control, lowering the kettlebell back down between your legs with a hip hinge.

Safety Considerations

Don't sacrifice form for weight. Start with a lighter weight and focus on proper technique.

Maintain a strong core engagement throughout the movement.

Don't pull the kettlebell too high above your head.

The Power of Progressive Overload

As you master these swing variations, the concept of progressive overload becomes crucial. This simply means gradually increasing the difficulty of your workouts over time. Here's how to implement it safely:

Increase Weight: Once you can comfortably perform a certain number of repetitions (e.g., 10-12) with good form, it's time to increase the weight of the kettlebell.

Increase Sets: Another way to progressively overload is to add additional sets of each variation to your workout routine.

Decrease Rest Periods: As your strength improves, you can shorten the rest periods between sets, keeping your workout challenging and efficient.

These presses work various muscle groups, including your shoulders, chest, triceps, and core, helping you develop a strong and sculpted upper body.

1. Two-Handed Push Press

The two-handed push press is a fantastic exercise for building upper body power and core stability. It combines the squat movement with a forceful overhead press, engaging multiple muscle groups.

How to Do It

Stand with your feet shoulder-width apart, holding the kettlebell with a two-handed grip (thumbs wrapped around the outside of the handle) at chest level. Keep your core engaged and back straight.

Hinge at your hips as if you're going to sit down in a chair, bending your knees slightly. This is the "dip" phase.

Explosively push back up through your heels, driving yourself upwards and simultaneously pressing the kettlebell overhead until your arms are straight. Imagine reaching for the ceiling with the kettlebell.

Lower the kettlebell back down to chest level with control, reversing the movement by hinging at your hips again.

Safety Considerations

Don't use your back to lift the kettlebell. The power comes from your legs and hips.

Keep your core engaged throughout the movement to protect your spine.

Don't lock your knees at the top of the movement. Maintain a slight bend.

Don't push the kettlebell behind your head. Keep it in line with your body.

2. Arnold Press

The Arnold press adds a rotational element to the traditional shoulder press, making it a more functional exercise that mimics everyday movements. It works your shoulders from multiple angles, promoting strength and stability.

How to Do It

Stand with your feet shoulder-width apart, holding a kettlebell in each hand with a neutral grip (thumbs wrapped around the outside of the handle). Your palms should be facing your body.

As you lift the kettlebells, begin by rotating your forearms outwards, so your palms face forward at the top of the movement (thumbs pointing upwards). This is the "winding" phase.

Press the kettlebells overhead until your arms are straight, keeping your core engaged and back straight.

Reverse the movement by lowering the kettlebells with control, rotating your forearms back to the starting position (palms facing your body) as you descend.

Safety Considerations

Start with lighter weights to ensure proper form.

Keep your core engaged throughout the movement to protect your spine.

Don't push the kettlebells behind your head. Keep them in line with your body.

Focus on controlled movements, avoiding any jerking or swinging.

3. Shoulder Press

The shoulder press is a traditional strength training exercise that effectively targets your shoulders. It's a fantastic way to build strength and definition in your upper body, especially when performed with proper form.

How to Do It

Stand with your feet shoulder-width apart, holding a kettlebell in each hand with a neutral grip (thumbs wrapped around the outside of the handle) at shoulder height. Your elbows should be bent at a 90-degree angle, with the kettlebells close to your body. Keep your core engaged and back straight.

Press the kettlebells straight overhead until your arms are fully extended. Squeeze your shoulder blades together at the top of the movement.

Lower the kettlebells back down to shoulder height with control, maintaining a 90-degree bend in your elbows.

Safety Considerations

Don't use momentum to lift the kettlebells. Focus on controlled movements.

Keep your core engaged throughout the movement to protect your spine.

Don't push the kettlebells behind your head. Keep them in line with your body.

Maintain a neutral spine with your back straight throughout the press.

Progression for Strength Gains

As you master these press variations and your strength improves, you can gradually increase the difficulty of your workouts. Here are some safe and effective ways to progress:

Increase Weight: Once you can comfortably perform a certain number of repetitions (e.g., 10-12) with good form, it's time to increase the weight of the kettlebells.

Increase Sets: Another way to progressively overload is to add additional sets of each press variation to your workout routine.

Decrease Rest Periods: As your strength improves, you can shorten the rest periods between sets, keeping your workout challenging and efficient.

4

Nutrition for Active Seniors

DIETARY NEEDS FOR SENIORS

As we grow older, taking care of our bodies becomes more important than ever. One of the best ways to do this is by eating a balanced diet. Let's talk about why this matters so much for seniors.

First off, a balanced diet helps us stay healthy as we age. It gives our bodies the right mix of nutrients to keep our muscles strong, our bones sturdy, our minds sharp, and our energy levels up. Plus, eating well can help us steer clear of common health problems like heart disease, diabetes, and osteoporosis.

But it's not just about preventing illness. A balanced diet also boosts our immune system, which is our body's defense against germs and sickness. By fueling up on the right foods, we can give our immune system the tools it needs to fight off infections and keep us feeling our best.

And let's not forget about energy. Eating a balanced diet provides us with the fuel we need to tackle our daily activities with gusto. Whether it's going for a walk, doing household chores, or spending time with loved ones, having enough energy makes it all easier and more enjoyable.

So, what exactly does a balanced diet look like? It's all about getting the right mix of different types of nutrients. For starters, we need protein to keep our muscles strong and help our bodies repair themselves. Good sources of protein include things like meat, fish, eggs, beans, and nuts.

Carbohydrates are another key part of the equation. They're our body's main source of energy, so we need to make sure we're getting enough of them. Healthy sources of carbs include whole grains like brown rice and whole wheat bread, as well as fruits, vegetables, and legumes.

And then there are fats. Yes, fats! They might have a bad reputation, but the truth is, our bodies need them too. Healthy fats, like the ones found in olive oil, avocados, and nuts, are important for things like absorbing vitamins and keeping our brains healthy.

But it's not just about the big stuff. We also need to pay attention to the little things – vitamins and minerals. These tiny nutrients play a big role in keeping our bodies running smoothly. For example, vitamin D helps our bodies absorb calcium, which keeps our bones strong. We can get vitamin D from things like sunlight and fortified foods. And then there's vitamin B12, which is important for our nerves and our blood. It's found in foods like meat, fish, and dairy products. And don't forget about vitamin C, which helps us fight off infections. You can get plenty of vitamin C from fruits and veggies like oranges, strawberries, and bell peppers.

Minerals are important too. Calcium is crucial for our bones and our muscles, so we need to make sure we're getting enough of it. You can find calcium in foods like milk, yogurt, and leafy greens. And then there's magnesium, potassium, and iron – all of which play important roles in keeping our bodies healthy and functioning properly.

So, how can we make sure we're eating a balanced diet? It's actually pretty simple. Try to eat a variety of different foods every day, including plenty of fruits, vegetables, whole grains, lean proteins, and healthy fats. Drink plenty of water too – staying hydrated is key to feeling good and staying healthy.

And if you're ever unsure about what to eat or how to make healthy choices, don't be afraid to ask for help. A registered dietitian can give you personalized advice and help you come up with a plan that works for you.

In the end, eating a balanced diet isn't just about staying healthy – it's about living your best life. By fueling your body with the right nutrients, you can feel great, stay active, and enjoy all the things that make life worth living. So go ahead, grab that apple or whip up a delicious salad – your body will thank you for it!

PREPARING AND RECOVERING WITH NUTRITION

When it comes to optimizing your exercise routine, what you eat before and after your workout can play a crucial role in your performance and recovery.

Before you embark on your workout, it's essential to provide your body with the right nutrients to fuel your efforts and maximize your performance. Here's what you need to know:

Pre-workout nutrition primes your body for activity by supplying the energy and nutrients necessary to sustain your efforts and optimize your performance. It can help enhance endurance, improve focus, and reduce the risk of fatigue and injury during exercise.

Focus on consuming a balanced combination of carbohydrates, protein, and healthy fats before your workout. Complex carbohydrates like whole grains, fruits, and vegetables provide a steady source of energy, while lean protein sources such as chicken, fish, or Greek yogurt support muscle repair and growth. Healthy fats from sources like nuts, seeds, or avocado can provide sustained energy and promote satiety during your workout.

Ideally, aim to eat a balanced meal or snack containing carbs, protein, and a small amount of fat approximately 1-3 hours before your workout. This timing allows your body to digest and absorb nutrients effectively, providing sustained energy throughout your exercise session.

After you've completed your workout, it's indispensable to refuel your body and support muscle recovery to ensure optimal performance and progress. Here's how you can promote recovery with post-workout nutrition:

Post-workout nutrition replenishes glycogen stores, restores electrolyte balance, and provides the building blocks necessary for muscle repair and growth. Consuming the right nutrients after exercise can help reduce muscle soreness, accelerate recovery, and enhance overall performance during subsequent workouts.

Focus on consuming a combination of protein and carbohydrates after your workout to promote muscle repair and glycogen replenishment. Lean protein sources like chicken, eggs, or a protein shake provide essential amino acids for muscle recovery, while fast-digesting carbohydrates like fruit or white rice facilitate glycogen restoration.

7-DAY MEAL PLAN TAILORED FOR SENIORS

Day 1

Breakfast:

Scrambled eggs with spinach and mushrooms.

Whole grain toast with avocado slices.

A cup of mixed berries.

Lunch:

Turkey and vegetable stir-fry with brown rice.

Side salad with mixed greens, cherry tomatoes, and balsamic vinaigrette.

Dinner:

Baked salmon with lemon and dill.

Quinoa pilaf with roasted vegetables (such as carrots, broccoli, and bell peppers).

Steamed asparagus spears.

A serving of Greek yogurt with honey for dessert.

Day 2

Breakfast:

Greek yogurt parfait with granola and sliced peaches.

Whole grain English muffin with almond butter.

Lunch:

Chickpea and vegetable soup.

Whole grain crackers with hummus.

Sliced melon for dessert.

Dinner:

Grilled chicken breast with rosemary.

Sweet potato mash.

Steamed green beans.

A slice of whole grain bread.

Mixed berries with a dollop of whipped cream for dessert.

Day 3

Breakfast:

Oatmeal topped with sliced bananas and chopped walnuts.

Hard-boiled egg on the side.

Lunch:

Quinoa salad with cucumber, tomato, and feta cheese.

Whole grain pita bread with tzatziki.

Sliced pineapple for dessert.

Dinner:

Beef and vegetable kebabs with a yogurt marinade.

Brown rice pilaf.

Steamed broccoli florets.

A serving of cottage cheese with fresh berries for dessert.

Day 4

Breakfast:

Whole grain pancakes with blueberry compote.

Turkey sausage links.

Lunch:

Tuna salad wrap with lettuce and tomato in a whole wheat tortilla.

Carrot and celery sticks with hummus.

Sliced mango for dessert.

Dinner:

Lentil curry with basmati rice.

Garlic sautéed spinach.

A slice of whole grain bread.

Baked apple with cinnamon for dessert.

Day 5

Breakfast:

Vegetable omelette with peppers, onions, and spinach.

Whole grain toast with avocado spread.

Lunch:

Chicken Caesar salad with whole grain croutons.

Whole grain crackers with cheese.

Sliced kiwi for dessert.

Dinner:

Baked cod with a lemon herb crust.

Quinoa salad with roasted vegetables.

Steamed green beans.

A serving of yogurt with sliced strawberries for dessert.

Day 6

Breakfast:

Smoothie made with spinach, banana, Greek yogurt, and almond milk.

Whole grain muffin.

Lunch:

Caprese salad with tomato, mozzarella, and basil.

Whole grain breadsticks.

Sliced peach for dessert.

Dinner:

Turkey meatloaf with a tomato glaze.

Mashed cauliflower.

Steamed carrots.

A serving of fruit salad with a dollop of Greek yogurt for dessert.

Day 7

Breakfast:

Whole grain waffles with fresh strawberries and a drizzle of maple syrup.

Turkey bacon strips.

Lunch:

Vegetable quinoa bowl with roasted chickpeas and tahini dressing.

Whole grain crackers with hummus.

Sliced pear for dessert.

Dinner:

Grilled shrimp skewers with pineapple and bell peppers.

Brown rice pilaf with peas.

Steamed broccoli florets.

A serving of cottage cheese with sliced peaches for dessert.

CONCLUSION

We believe this guide has empowered you to unlock your inner strength and potential. If you found the information valuable and enjoyed your reading experience, please consider leaving a positive review and rating for this book. Your feedback helps us reach more seniors who are ready to embrace an active lifestyle.

So, keep swinging, keep pressing, and keep striving for a healthier, more vibrant you! May your kettlebell journey be filled with strength, accomplishment, and a newfound sense of empowerment.

Made in United States
Cleveland, OH
05 February 2025

14103740R00039